Wedding

Planning for

Spoonies

Meara Bartlett

ISBN:

ISBN-13: 978-1-7363736-0-6

To my wonderful spouse Tyson:

Writing this book has been an epic love letter to you that each time I sit down to write it, I am reminded of the joy it is to be your wife.

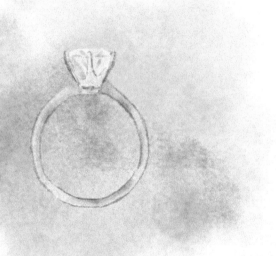

Introduction

Table of Contents

1. Introduction Letter 1

2. What is a Spoonie? 5

3. Meet Our Spoonies 7

4. The Engagement 11

5. Define Your Vision 17

6. Planning Timeline 23

7. To DIY or Not to DIY? 31

8. The Beginning 33

    a. Wedding Planning 101 35

    b. My Planning Story 37

    c. The Budget 39

    d. The Guest List 46

9. The Vendors 51

    a. Contracts 53

    b. The Venue 57

    c. Photography & Videography 67

    d. Flowers 70

    e. Invitations 73

    f. Choosing the Wedding Party 77

    g. Hotel Blocks 80

h. Wedding Planners & Others...................................... 82

i. Wedding Clothes.. 84

j. Flower Girls, Ring Bearer, and Pets 98

k. Refreshments.. 100

    i. Caterer & Baker 100

    ii. Drinks.. 103

l. Music... 104

m. Cosmetologists 108

n. Transportation 109

o. Rentals... 111

10. The Extras 113

a. Décor.. 115

b. Favors & Gifts.. 118

c. Premarital Counseling.. 119

11. Accommodations for Yourself and Your Guests................. 121

12. The Wedding Day 133

a. Day-Of Timeline 135

b. Order of Ceremony 138

13. Planning with Your Disabled Partner................................ 141

14. Thank You for Reading 151

Introduction: Why I Wrote This Book

In June 2019, one of my dreams came true – the man of my dreams proposed to me. But our journey together didn't come without challenges after I said "yes." In July 2019, I was sent to the ER for severe, unrelenting pain that lasted one week. The doctor said I most likely had nerve damage. I mourned this new chapter of my life. However, my then-fiancé entirely embraced this "new me." Expressing concern for me, he fed me in bed, saw that my medications were managed, and held my hand by my bedside while I cried. He had unwavering love for me.

I never expected to experience such love from a person. Today he still is my rock, and I can be my chaotic self. Oftentimes I wondered what I did to deserve it. I frequently asked him why he still wanted to be with me, and he responded that he liked having me around. My husband loves me for me. I can't ask for a bigger blessing.

Developing intense, chronic, physical pain is taxing on the person with it and everyone involved. I experienced anger toward my situation and directed it at pretty much everyone around me. But my future husband stayed. He remained gentle and kind, despite all my emotional episodes as well as my physical ones.

I was still bedridden during the month of my wedding, and my fiancé and I were contemplating cancelling the honeymoon. Seeking to empower me with new tools for my new life, he ordered me a cream and silver sparkly cane with a hooked handle. Its shimmery appearance was to make me feel better about having to use a mobility aid and to get me through the honeymoon and wedding day.

The sparkliness of the cane streaked straight down the walking part and curled in little pearls on the handle. It did empower me. Glitter is my jet fuel and I'm the kind of girl who rocks face glitter to go to the grocery store. Now I could go to the grocery store, and I did so in a blaze of glitter and sophistication.

No canes were needed on my wedding day, as we had an emergency wedding at my parents' house. Thanks to moving the wedding inside my parents' house, I was able to take breaks and hide from guests if needed. It was also a much smaller area than my original 300-acre venue, where I would have to cross a bridge and part of a forest.

I became a disabled bride. During my wedding planning process, I learned a lot and wanted to pass it on. I also wanted to show other brides that there are many tools for them out there, so this book is full of research, as well as my own personal experience.

Planning a wedding can feel lonely when you are disabled or chronically ill and I wish to be your fairy guide to help you through your process. In part your need for this is due to not knowing where to look, who to talk to, or who is in your circle. Online there are many resources and groups to hook up to, such as Offbeatbride.com, where I have written about my experiences before, and TheMighty.com. These websites are wonderful and I do love them. But I questioned why disabled couples were sequestered off to certain corners of the Internet and not brought out into more light. We deserve to be seen, and we deserve a book.

You and your partner aren't the only ones out there,

Meara Bartlett

What is a Spoonie?

Some of you may have picked up this book wondering what on Earth a spoonie is. The term spoonie comes from Christine Miserandino's essay "The Spoon Theory" where she explains her chronic illness, lupus, by taking spoons away from her roommate at a restaurant to demonstrate how she has to ration out energy during her day and can't get any back. She shows how a person who is disabled may have to be very careful with the tasks they choose to do during their day to prevent burnout, a symptom flare, or the danger of passing out. You can be disabled, chronically ill, and a spoonie all at the same time, or just one, depending on what you choose to call yourself or whether your specific condition is physically taxing or not. There will be more discussion about what a spoonie is later in the book.

Meet Our Spoonies

Throughout this book, you will see quotes sprinkled in. These are from a group of people who volunteered to contribute their experiences to this book to further its depth and to help you. I hope you might identify with some of them. They are not diagnosed with the entire list of conditions covered in this book.

Here I asked them: "What is your condition and explain how it affects your daily life." I wanted you all to understand the context in which they will be answering questions throughout the book. It's important to know where someone is coming from to understand their needs, and how they might encourage you. Now, let's meet the contributors below.

Carrie-Ann says not to miss a minute of your wedding day. "I have cerebral palsy which means that I use a wheelchair. I'm unable to walk but am able to transfer from one chair to another. I also have many experiences of anxiety and depression, and PTSD. At the time that I got married I was struggling with severe social anxiety." She was married in 2012 to her long-time boyfriend.

At the time Rachel was married, she was housebound. She suffers from "fibromyalgia and myalgia encephalitis, AKA chronic fatigue [in addition to] chronic migraines roughly 28 days a month. This involves chronic, ongoing full-body pain, as well as extreme fatigue, and becoming easily exhausted. I use a walking stick to help with this." She married her husband Fred in June of 2000.

Fred has epilepsy, which he developed after his wedding to Rachel. "He has tonic-clinic seizures, which are what you think of when you picture a seizure, falling to the ground, uncontrolled shaking. He also has focal seizures, where he loses consciousness but it is not always obvious, as he may just look like he is daydreaming or not paying attention." He also has depression and anxiety. Looking at the numbers though, Fred and Rachel have been married for 20 years!

Meagan suffers from a rare, painful disease that is linked to having had colon cancer at a young age called familial adenomatous polyposis due to it causing the presence of many polyps. She also has another disease, short bowel syndrome. "Short bowel syndrome is a rare disease that is caused by the removal of or dysfunction of part or all of the small intestine and/or large intestine. This can cause life-threatening malnutrition and dehydration," she said of how it directly impacted her in more than one way. For her wedding, Meagan wore her grandmother's dress and a handmade mantilla veil. She did not have symptoms on her day.

Amy has a chronic illness known as hypermobile Ehlers-Danlos syndrome (hEDs). "For me, it means that I manage a lot of leg, hip, and neck pain and my ribs and vertebrae subluxate frequently (less frequently after a year of physical therapy!). I'm fortunate in that I don't dislocate at all and have done enough strength training that I do not require bracing of any joints. My hEDs really affects my gut, which affects my skin a lot, so I am constantly watching my diet to avoid trigger foods that could cause gut issues and acne or eczema. Stress management is crucial for me too because any stressors (good or bad) will trigger pain, gut and skin flares." Her ceremony was down-to-earth, personal, and touching. This kept her stress low and her flares away.

K. W. Warburton had friends who accommodated her during the planning process when no one else would. "I have postural orthostatic tachycardia syndrome (POTS), which is a condition that causes dizzy spells, chronic fatigue, and a fast heart rate. These symptoms mainly occur when you are standing up (hence the postural part) and those with POTS fall onto a spectrum with regards to the severity of their condition. I have a very severe form of POTS that left me bedridden for several years." K. W. Warburton met her partner at school, where he stood by her side when she was diagnosed with POTS.

Each of these people, fueled with love for themselves and someone else, dreamed up a wedding day. Dreaming is the most important part of the wedding planning. It's also called a vision. They saw through their visions to give them their perfect wedding day. But before they made it to that point, they had to become engaged.

Where it All Begins: The Engagement

Engagements look different for everyone. Some of you may be engaged, but don't have rings on your fingers. Others of you might just be dreaming of when that sparkly diamond is finally placed on your hand one summer evening and you're whisked away to white dresses and wedded bliss! There is nothing wrong with either of these scenarios. Or maybe you're reading this out of pure curiosity. Perhaps you're a wedding planner and you're dealing with a newly engaged disabled couple wanting to learn more. Maybe you saw this and have a disabled friend who is recently engaged and thought this would make an appropriate present.

Whoever you are, you know somewhere someone decided that they should marry somebody sometime, whether that's you, your partner, your parents, a friend, or a client. Usually this does involve a ring at some point – whether the couple picks it out together at a jewelry store, it's custom designed, someone gets down on one knee, or a combination of these, your ring is gorgeous and priceless. Likewise, your engagement is perfect and an irreplaceable moment in time because it starts you down the path to matrimony.

However, there is an art to spreading the word about your engagement. You're probably filled with joy and want the whole world to know you've found your person – but exercise caution before posting that picture on social media. Call your mom first, then your siblings, then best friends. And understand that who knows what will tell someone else next, and feelings can get hurt depending on who gets a phone call when. It's much better to call than to text when it comes to announcing your engagement. Once the important phone calls are done, then you can post across your social media platforms. Going the virtual route first can seem a bit cold to your friends and family.

If you have children, they should absolutely be the first to know, all rules aside. They are gaining a new parent, possibly new siblings, and their worlds are changing in a huge way. Communicate with them as clearly and delicately as possible what this means in their family context in person.

Should you have children with a previous partner or spouse, contact your ex over the phone and as cordially as possible let them know the news first, regardless of your relationship. This is to avoid your child from gushing to your ex-partner and speculating before you can arrange to talk first. Even if you don't have children with an ex-spouse, it is a good idea to let them know the news before posting on social media.

You have the option of an engagement party. If your parents are willing to host it, they may be willing to foot the bill. Either or both of your parents can host. These days, most couples host the engagement party themselves and pay. If you can't afford this, don't worry. It isn't an absolute must. Should you go this route, invite your close family and friends to announce your engagement. Don't worry about formal invitations – you can send invites via email, or a simple white card with text in the mail stating that "Alex Doe is Engaged to Taylor Smith."

The standard engagement is a year. You can plan a beautiful wedding in days or weeks – I had family friends who planned a pretty waterfront wedding in three days. While in wedding planning, rules are more like guidelines, it's still good practice to plan it in a year, as the golden rule to reduce stress.

Family Affairs

Sometimes, families aren't always gracious when they hear about a betrothal, especially one to a disabled person, or an able-bodied person. Almost always the root of it all is a sense of a lack of control or fear of change in their lives, and yes, sometimes unknown prejudice can be part of it. It isn't about you or your partner. Your parents are people and their behavior reflects on them. Should your family react negatively to your engagement, there is no need for your partner to hear it. Try to shield your partner and act like an adult, even if your parents aren't.

Don't tolerate disrespect from your family toward yourself or your partner. Express that by saying that by them hurting you or your partner, your family is hurting a part of yourself. Whether or not this works doesn't really matter, but it does protect you and your partner's dignity, and you can rest better at night than your family by being the guilt-free, respectable adult.

However, your partner will eventually find out about your family's dislike. Have a "just the facts" conversation with your partner about your family drama. Only do this once, reassuring your partner that you love them wholeheartedly and will not let your family tear your relationship apart. Make sure to not bring your emotions to the table that aren't positive. The key here is not to vent, but inform.

Sometimes writing letters you never send and then ripping them up is a good way to vent stress toward others if the situation gets really tough on your mind. Family situations can be brutal and damaging. Protecting yourself and your partner may mean developing new coping skills. Invest in good self-care habits and find creative ways to vent to anyone (such as good, close friends who won't fib) but your partner when it comes to family matters.

It's possible that if you accidentally vent to your partner about how your family is upset that you're getting married, your partner might mistakenly see this as you breaking up with them. Regardless, this action might hurt your partner, and very naturally, your relationship.

Define Your Vision

Why you should have a wedding vision: it makes the rest of the planning easier if you do it first!

Let's daydream! Maybe you've kept a box under your bed of wedding magazine clippings since you were 12. Or you savored a game of M*A*S*H more than the rest of your classmates, especially the M part. Perhaps you have a lingering secret Pinterest board dying to debut, or it has proudly been on display since 2011. This could also all sound disgusting to you.

Whether or not you did or didn't dream about your wedding your entire life, it's time to start brainstorming. It's your wedding. I guarantee you will have opinions about it once wedding planning begins, no matter how much you may object to country clubs and prefer courthouses. That's a brainstorm to begin with!

Begin brainstorming by owning it. Your wedding is, well, *yours*. This is your once in a lifetime with this one person who decided they loved you. Ultimately, it's a big party!

17

Did you just recoil at the term party? Or did you relish the image of a crowded room, where everyone there is here to see you?

That's Step #1: how do I like to keep company?

Next let's figure out where and how you spend your time. Are you outdoorsy? Or are you more likely to stay inside reading? That might mean a library wedding is in order. Perhaps you enjoy painting and would love to perform matrimony at an altar in an art gallery. If you'd rather be studying scripture, a traditional house of worship venue with heavy religious motifs is likely your pick.

What are a few of your favorite things? Are you geeky or more English garden? Perhaps geeky *and* English garden? Which dance do you prefer: the Lindy Hop or Copperhead Road? What suits *your* vibe?

Step #2 is: what are my hobbies and interests?

Collaborate with your partner and go over your mutual interests and hobbies. Where do you go to spend time having fun together? What are your values? Did you meet in Kindergarten and bond early together playing sports at the town rec center, or did you meet after college and bond over board games?

Include your partner and make a list of where and what you do together. Go by estimated percentages. Maybe look at pictures on your phone – where they were taken, or even memes you've sent each other.

Step #3 is: what do I like to drink?

This somewhat ties back to Step #1. Do you drink and do your friends and family drink? How much do you drink and under what circumstances? Are you a beer can or a wine glass? Do you not drink at all for health reasons?

These questions will help you determine another aspect of how you might interact with your guests. Don't judge yourself for wanting an open bar or no bar at all. This is your day, and no one can ruin it for you but your peace of mind. Here's a toast to your serenity!

Imagination Determination:

The vision is one of the most fun parts of wedding planning. Maybe you've had a vision your entire life! Whether you have or not, now is the time to let your imagination run wild. Think about what you're a fan of! "I wanted a fun, short ceremony so we had a Blues Brothers themed wedding. The men dressed as the Blues Brothers. The ring bearer had a briefcase handcuffed to him and wore Converse shoes (like in Blues Brothers 2). Everyone danced down the aisle to Blues Brothers music instead of walking down the aisle. My then husband and I were handcuffed to each other when we were pronounced married." This was Meagan's vision, taken from movies and activities she enjoyed. It resulted in a unique, fun experience. You could do something similar, or go the traditional route. Maybe a little bit of both?

Staying true to your vision can be a bit of an adventure. Sometimes staying true to yourself can prove challenging to those around you. But your vision truly is the most important part of wedding planning – just remember that and keep it in the back of your mind throughout the process.

Your Vision Is a Quest

Wedding planning is an action-romance-comedy-thriller film. It's primarily a film because of all the visuals, and a thriller because of all the twists and turns. It's fast-paced at times, and slow with tense suspense. Sometimes there's a funny anecdote or two. But at the heart is the romance that fuels your vision for the wedding.

Much like any good film, a wedding vision requires some creativity. You don't need to be a Picasso to plan a wedding, all you need to do is think outside the box a little bit to figure out how to get from point A to B using calligraphic flourishes instead of a straight line. Or binary code. In wedding planning you seek and find: that's what makes it a quest.

For example, let's say you fall in love with a mermaid-themed library wedding. Or a classy chateau affair. These two are your "seeks," or your quests to embark on. But you only have $5000. Now we'll set forth on our journey.

Mermaid library wedding? No problem, financially speaking. Classy chateau? Problem? No, not if you're willing to think outside the box. If a friend or relative of yours has a nice home, see if you can use it for the weekend. Thrift or borrow fine china, and decorate to your heart's content. With a little imagination and ingenuity, you can transform that house into your chateau.

Or you could rent a luxury house for the weekend and bring thrifted decorations. As long as the location is nice and there's plenty of space for your guests, you can have your maison dream destination. It's the same concept, only this time you're overstepping encroaching on a friendship to get your dream wedding.

It's okay if there are challenges along the way. Maybe your future in-laws think mermaids and libraries aren't classy enough for *their* child's wedding. But your partner loves books and their favorite childhood movie involves mermaids. You both love libraries and mermaids. Remember your marvelous vision and hold true to it, because this is your wedding.

Planning Timeline

If you're wondering how exactly to plan and when, here is a rough outline – a guideline – to direct you and inspire you along your journey. This serves as a helpful roadmap to show you the ropes to wedding planning. Don't get stressed if you veer off course. This isn't word of law. Simply refer back to this timeline if you need a little help with what next steps you could take in your planning.

12 Month Timeline

Here is a 12-month timeline. Some of this can be moved around – let's say, when you hire a wedding planner or coordinator based on how experienced they are and if they are with a company – but for the most part, some vendors are better off hired first, such as a photographer and a venue.

Notice that in a disability-friendly timeline, the couple collects addresses and sends invitations as soon as the venue is found in order to gather data from your guests.

12-11 months

Create vision

Find venue

Set date

Begin research

Book photographer & videographer

Book florist

Collect addresses and send invitations

Start registry

9-6 months

Choose wedding party

Reserve hotel blocks

Hire wedding day coordinator or planner

Order wedding dress

Book caterer

Book baker

Create playlist

Book musicians

Book cosmetologists

Book transportation

Book rentals: include linens

Book rehearsal dinner

Begin DIY day-of signage (menus, seating chart, programs, etc.)

6-4 months

Order signage if you aren't DIY-ing

Make detailed lists of:

Photography shot lists and send to your photographer

Menus

Create floral design and send to florist

Draft timelines for the day-of

Make honeymoon reservations & check passports

Learn what the marriage license requirements are for your area

4-1 Months

Have dress fitted 1 month out, keep trying on the dress about every week

Obtain marriage license (in some states the license is only good for 8 weeks, so be careful!)

Plan ceremony

Attend premarital counseling

Purchase wedding rings

1-2 Weeks Before

Confirm guest list

Confirm day-of transportation

Shop and pack for honeymoon

Book sound system if DIY

Put final cash payments for vendors in labeled envelopes

2-3 Days Before

Confirm transportation to the airport for your honeymoon

Organize day-of emergency kit

Have wedding dress steamed

Contact venues

Determine order of your attendants

Confirm order with florist

Confirm wedding transportation with your driver

Day Before

Get manicure and pedicure (if you wish)

Have ceremony rehearsal

Pass off marriage license to officiant

Give attendants their gifts at rehearsal dinner

6-Month Timeline

You can still get everything done in less time. I know I did. Here is an altered timeline of when to get what done when in order.

6-4 months

Find venue

Set date

Create vision

Begin research

Collect addresses and send invitations

Book photographer & videographer

Order wedding dress

Book florist

Choose wedding party

Reserve hotel blocks

Hire wedding day coordinator or planner

Book caterer

Book baker

Book rentals: include linens

Book rehearsal dinner

Check passport status

Start registry

Begin DIY day-of signage (menus, seating chart, programs, etc.)

4-2 months

Order signage if you aren't DIY-ing

Make detailed lists of:

Photography shot lists and send to your photographer

Menus

Create playlist

Book musicians

Book cosmetologists

Book transportation

Compile flower display list and send to florist

Draft timelines for the day-of

Make honeymoon reservations

Learn what the marriage license requirements are for your area

2-1 Months

Have dress fitted 1 month out, keep trying on the dress about every week

Obtain marriage license (in some states the license is only good for 8 weeks, so be careful!)

Attend premarital counseling

Purchase wedding rings

Plan ceremony

1-2 Weeks Before

Confirm guest list

Confirm day-of transportation

Shop and pack for honeymoon

Book sound system if DIY

Put final cash payments for vendors in labeled envelopes

2-3 Days Before

Confirm transportation to the airport for your honeymoon

Organize day-of emergency kit

Have wedding dress steamed

Contact venues

Figure out order of your attendants

Confirm order with florist

Confirm wedding transportation with your driver

Day Before

Get manicure and pedicure (if you wish)

Have ceremony rehearsal

Pass off marriage license to officiant

Give attendants their gifts at rehearsal dinner

To DIY or Not to DIY?

Weddings are team sports and people love happy occasions. Your friends and family are going to want to help you. Let them help! Host a DIY crafting party with your friends. Weddings are about love, and you deserve love from your community!

It can be easy to see help as infantilizing – and it may appear as a fine line. Having your vision in mind and setting boundaries with the wedding vision rather than experiencing what you perceive as a slight by someone donating Christmas lights or tulle can help you do a check on whether or not someone really perceives you as less capable. Even able-bodied people need help DIY-ing, that's why wedding planners exist and largely cater to able-bodied couples! Just know what your boundaries are with the vision. If someone tries to veer you off course with their help, you know they've overstepped and really aren't helping. Have a talk with them and see if they can be corrected.

I completely DIY'd my wedding while recently diagnosed. For the DIY route, consider a day-of coordinator to help with logistics the day-of. For those with less DIY savvy, definitely consider a full-service wedding planner. You may save money in the long run with a good, experienced wedding planner.

The best day-of coordinators will be extremely supportive, especially when you reveal you have a condition. Mine was. The only problem was my date moved into the week and I lost her due to scheduling. She had a day job. Look for a full-time wedding professional if you fear your wedding might fall into the danger-zone hijinks category.

The number one thing to look for in any wedding planner or day-of coordinator is intelligence, followed by empathy. If your wedding planner's website proclaims they are educated and organized, by all means book them! But not without meeting them and seeing them display their wit.

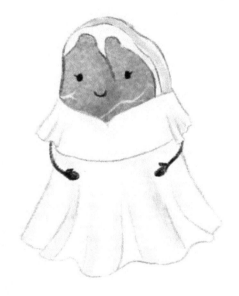

The Beginning

Wedding Planning 101

How exactly do you plan a wedding?

One step at a time. Amy suffers from exaggerated symptoms when stressed. She landed on a charming backyard wedding to avoid feeling ill. With a more relaxed setting, she was able to focus more on the details that mattered to her. This leads me back to my first point: parcel out the wedding planning into little steps, like the ones outlined in this book, and give yourself time to execute them in order to avoid high levels of stress. If you're stressed out with a chronic illness, you can inflict physical pain as well as inner turmoil if you don't take wedding planning one day at a time, one parcel at a time.

Let's say you decide you need a caterer. You could designate one day for two hours of research over the weekend. Come up with a spreadsheet of contact information and dietary information. Make this the one thing you do that day for the allotted time. Stay organized in your spreadsheet, and you'll be golden. Simply allot enough time to be serene and stress-free.

Please try not to plan everything at once. I know it's easy to think you're crunched for time. Some people plan their weddings in one month, and they are just as married! Perfection is not the goal of a wedding. It's true love and happiness. As long as you have that, you're golden. Just remember not to hurry love. It will be waiting for you at the end of the aisle.

Your love will be there for you, whether you sense it or not. The whole reason you are planning this wedding is because you are loved. Feel this love for yourself and your partner. There is joy to be found in all the little details of planning, and of course, the even greater joy of your wedding day.

Focus on the goal of a celebration of love. You are declaring your love for your partner in front of someone or a group of people. This isn't the time to be dizzying about who to impress. And this ultimately isn't about you, either. It's about fun!

If this kind of fun stresses you out, think about simple ways to express your love the way Amy did. A day of worry isn't worth anything. But a day of joy is worth the world.

My Planning Story

I planned two weddings to one man. My first wedding was full-on, hard-hitting planning, with spreadsheets, dreams, and Pinterest boards spanning months. I designed menus, printed my own invitations, and called caterers. From day one I was meeting with florists and researching cake bakers. (PS: do you know how hard it is to find a vegan cake baker in Texas that's affordable?)

The first three months of my engagement were like a race. All I did was wedding plan. I had a tiny budget, I was going to stay inside it, and I did. My wedding was going to be the classiest budget wedding the world ever saw. In my humble opinion, I'm proud to say that it was. This might be because of how dedicated I was to my almost completely DIY wedding.

But then, my plans were washed away by mobility issues. I couldn't access my venue with a cane. I now had to plan a wedding in 48 hours. And I did it.

Frantically ordering off of Amazon and redesigning a seating chart, I was going to ensure this wedding was just as classy, hopefully more, than my original jazz country forest wedding. Because I had disclosed my health problems to my vendors earlier, I magically kept all of them but the day-of coordinator. The only reason she could not come was because she had a day job that kept her from working weekdays.

With the help of my family, we completely DIY'd a Victorian wonderland in the beautiful Texas hill country. I had antique teacups and lace tablecloths. We repurposed decorations from the original wedding, and used heirlooms from around the house. The aisle runner arrived just as my husband and I were presented to our guests. But it was beautiful, and I did it in 48 hours.

If I could plan a dainty Victorian wedding in 48 hours, you can do anything.

The Budget

Everyone should allow room for personal emergencies when planning a wedding. Subsequently, I have included a basic budget outline and the Ultra-Lite Below $6k, which was my budget. I successfully pulled it off, and my wedding was beautiful.

Like all people, disabled people come at all income levels. Pick which one best suits you and your finances or use it as a guide to create your own. If you've been dying to put on a gala your whole life but are struggling financially, know you don't have to have tons of funds to do so. You could also have a long engagement to save up.

The Miscellaneous Category

As you will see, there is this mysterious "miscellaneous" category further on in the numbers portion of this chapter. Never fear! Life is random and it affects weddings, too. Think of it as your wedding's emergency fund, just as you have an emergency fund. Just try to have at least 1% of your wedding budget put away for hiccups, maybe more – such as a change in venue, or another vendor. An example I had was my unforeseen wedding dress alterations, followed by a second wedding dress, then having an unavailable original day-of coordinator and needing to hire a new one.

Basic Outline For a Wedding Budget	
Reception	55%
Ceremony	12%
Photography	10%
Wedding Planner	10%
Attire	8%
Miscellaneous	5%

This is a basic template for a wedding budget. You can take however much cash you have and apply it to these percentages to stay on point and not overflow into any categories. There are ways to reduce these percentages so you have more money to spend on other areas, or less to spend overall.

For example, you could get married at a free venue with a reception space to drastically reduce the cost of your ceremony and reception, and opt not to serve alcohol. You could invest this money into a nicer dress or hire a wedding planner. Or you could hit 0% in the wedding planner department by not hiring one at all.

My Budget: Ultra-Lite Below $6k Budget

Ultra-Lite Below $6k Budget	
Reception	42%
Photography:	23%
Attire	20%
Miscellaneous	15%
Ceremony	0%

Here is a more detailed, broken-down budget from the basic budget. This was my husband and my budget. As you can see, we didn't pay for many of the categories – entertainment, ceremony, or transportation, which resulted in gaps in the budget, as shown in the miscellaneous category. This meant we were free to spend money elsewhere.

This is because we were part of a community that supported us in large ways. We were gifted décor, allowed to borrow tables and chairs, and received discounts by shopping local. Our photographer actually gave us 50% off for having the venue be in the same small town as her because she was a busy new mom used to driving long distances to weddings. For those in other areas, consider hiring a college student as long as you like their portfolio.

We hit 0% in other categories by having free entertainment. Our free entertainment was an iPod DJ performed by a free Spotify student trial. We used my smartphone and the Spotify app. My father officiated the ceremony for free, and we used decorations gifted to us as well as what we already had for the ceremony space. We used white chairs from the church I grew up in for seating. For transportation, my maid of honor drove me around and my getaway car was my husband's Honda.

As for gifts, we scored 0% by being crafty. For wedding party gifts, my sister, who was my maid of honor, received a nice Christmas present instead of a wedding gift as we were married the week before Christmas. If you want to know how you can hit 0% in this category, you can. Other ways to be crafty and have free wedding favors and gifts include photocopying old family recipe cards, knitting potholders, painting a wedding party member a picture yourself, or handcrafted hobby jewelry.

Photos from my under $6,000 wedding

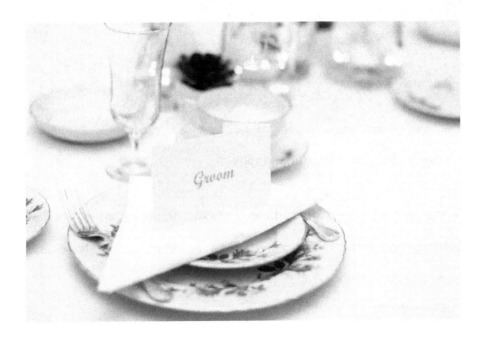

Photo Credit: Tauni Joy Photography. Heirloom pink and white floral china, gold-tone flatware and crystal drinkware. Perched on top of the triangular-folded napkin is a card with the word "Groom" in gold letters.

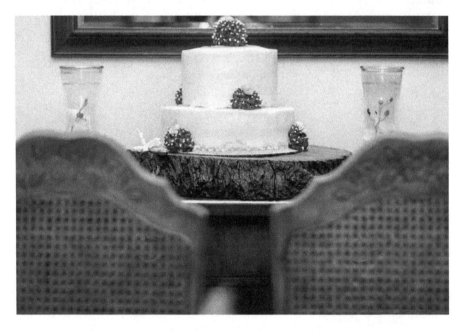

Photo Credit: Tauni Joy Photography

White cake with decorative edible green succulents on brown wooden heirloom credenza overlooking brown heirloom dining table and brown wicker chairs.

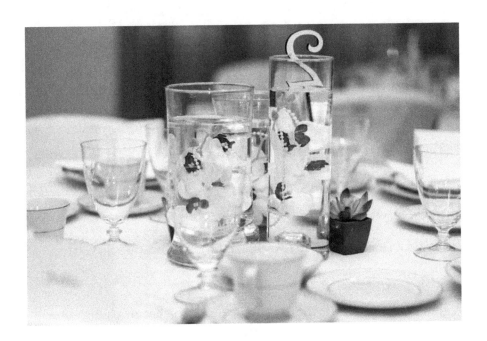

Photo Credit: Tauni Joy Photography

White and purple orchids submerged in water on a white tablecloth with vintage white teacup surrounded by shimmering crystal drinkware.

The Guest List

Now, don't skip over this part before going on to the Venue chapter. If you don't have a guest count, you won't know what venue size to get!

The guest list is the most debatable part of wedding planning. It's the most people-involved part of the process. Who do we offend? Who do we not offend? Do you really need to see those cousins in North Dakota you haven't seen since you were five although your mother wants you to?

A good rule of thumb is the two-year rule. If you haven't hung out with them personally on a one-to-one level outside of school, church, or work in the past two years, you don't have to send an invitation. Same applies to family, unless it's siblings, parents, and grandparents.

You are going to break eggs during this process. If you try to keep everybody happy, *you* will not be happy.

If you've got pain or an illness, you've probably got a short temper and want to be your best self on your special day. Be smart and surround yourself with only the people you like best. It's simple logic: if you feel bad, you might make other people feel bad, which will make you feel worse. If you feel bad, surround yourself with people who make you feel good, you will feel better and everyone will enjoy the day more.

Even for those who are disabled and do not experience pain, only inviting those who know what your disability is will put you at ease during the stress of the wedding. You will be more relaxed and less Godzilla on your special day if everyone in attendance has good familiarity with your disability.

Rachel and Fred had a guest list of 30 who were mostly family. Everyone knew about Rachel's disability, so she didn't have to pretend or be perceived as rude. She also had an entire wedding who looked after her.

Besides, you'll save money in the long run!

I do understand this will be difficult for some, especially for those coming from large, extended families or marrying into them. Just remember you're an adult, and you've come this far if you decide to cut down the guest list.

There are alternatives to drastically cutting the guest list for those with large, extended families – although getting there might feel uncomfortable. You can call or email everyone on the guest list disclosing your disability or illness. This can put you more at ease. It is up to your comfort level with your family or your partner's family. Or, propose the use of technology – similar to the way outlined in the next section – to include everyone together without them being physically present.

Guest Lists and Pandemics

Currently there is a limit on groups of 10 in the United States because of pandemic outbreaks. Who knows how long this will last. In light of this, I have written this segment. Please keep your in-person guest list small out of respect for their lives and yours.

Only invite your local friends and immediate family to come in-person, but only up to 10 including yourself, the officiant, your photographer, and your partner. Then, designate one person present to livestream the wedding via Facebook if you were intending on inviting a huge crowd, or Zoom if you wanted a more modest one. Lastly, send out virtual invitations with information regarding livestreaming, whether it be on Facebook Live or Zoom. You can do this through your wedding website, which will be discussed in later chapters.

80 vs 20: A Battle Over the Guest List

I come from an unusually small family. My parents are both only children, and I have one living grandparent. In my immediate family it's only my younger sister and myself.

On my husband's side of the family … well … He's fully stocked. His mother has 4 siblings and his father has 2. When it came time to create the guest list, my husband handed the guest list over to his mother and she invited everyone on their side.

Some of you may be thinking, so what? Just invite your friends. And I did invite my friends. But it wasn't enough to tip the scale where I could overcome my husband's family. But I did have another community I belonged to: my parents' church.

My father is a minister at a small country church I still volunteer at to this day. Both my sister and I refer to the church members as our pseudo-family, as we had no cousins, aunts, or uncles growing up. I decided that every person in the church directory was going to receive an invitation. Almost everyone RSVP'd, and one helped pay for my wedding dress. This bumped our guest list up to 80, and I was winning.

Then I got sick, and my parents moved the venue and reduced the guest list to 20. Everyone who came except two people were on my husband's side.

But at the same time, we were surrounded by people. The people who showed up on my side really, really cared – my old roommate helped with my makeup and a family friend helped run the wedding with my maid of honor. I don't know if just anyone would have been willing to work at a wedding. It made it just that bit more special.

It's best to lay your pride aside when it comes to the guest list and toss politics away. Invite who you love and accept your partner's family for who they are to the best of your abilities. Don't take disrespect, but disrespect is not a guest list. (Just tell your partner to take the reins and not give them to their mother.)

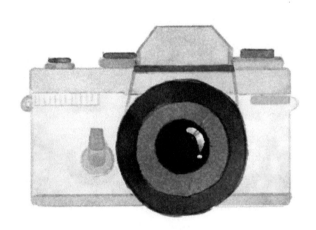

The Vendors

This chapter covers vendors, how to deal with them, and a loose timeline that follows the one earlier in the book.

Safety in Contracts

What if something goes wrong with your wedding day? What if a vendor goes belly-up? How do you ensure a vendor shows up on the wedding day?

I have four words: Get a signed contract.

How to go about this? Look online first. Scope out all photographers, venues, and other vendors on the web and make a spreadsheet. Look for ones that have blogs and social media. See when, if, and how they use pronouns. When you find one you feel comfortable with, negotiate over email instead of over the phone. Watch their wording with pronouns, such as whether they ask about your partner instead of your husband or fiancée.

When dealing with vendors over email, it's a good idea to have an email folder specifically for wedding-related tomfoolery. You can even have subfolders. An example would be Wedding – vendors – photography, or Wedding – wedding party – wedding attendants, or Wedding

– wedding party – in-laws. If you're a virtual planner instead of a paper planner, this is a great way to go. Although paper planning is fun, as our communications are progressing more and more digital, all of us have to get organized virtually at least a little bit.

Especially when it comes to disability, it's logical to be a digital planner. Conduct almost all inquiries online until you absolutely have to look at that one venue or taste that cake, then get a signed and dated copy of a contract. Take a picture of it with your phone if the situation needs. If you come across a vendor who doesn't do contracts after you ask for one do not pursue, or find your own copy of a wedding vendor contract online. This way, if someone tries to violate your rights, you can provide evidence that they did.

You can also make your own contract template or edit the contract on the following page.

Wedding Vendor Name Contract

Name of Client:

Phone:

Address:

Wedding Date:

This contract made on this day ___, between ___now called the wedding vendor and ____, now called the client. The contract shall be effective between _____ and _____.

The wedding vendor shall be responsible for the following services:

- List service here, such as wedding dress, venue

The wedding vendor will be paid in advance a sum of __ by the client for necessary preparations. After the completion of the wedding, the client must pay a sum of ___ for the vendor's services.

Signature of client:

Signature of wedding vendor:

When it comes to vendors, you can find the rest of your wedding dream team by asking the ones you have for suggestions – such as asking your florist for a DJ and vice versa. A good rule of thumb that you have good people on your side is that they never try to push your budget or complain about it, they simply make it work. For example, when you give your budget to your cake baker, they don't scoff or try to negotiate.

The Venue

As always, the vision comes first. What do you like to do? That should determine your wedding venue more than anything. Pretty much all venues can be made accessible. But once your theme is determined by your shared hobbies, values, and interests, you'll know where to go for your venue.

For example, let's talk about values for a second. Do you value dazzling your guests most or do you value your family and home faith more? This determines whether you'll go for a ritzy ballroom venue downtown or the house of worship you grew up in.

The venue is one of the most important aspects of the wedding. It starts off your wedding planning process and determines your wedding date. You should book it as soon as you get engaged, as some venues are booked two years out. Here I'm going to break it down by needs for what to keep in mind for a venue.

Do keep your guests in mind of all abilities, distances, and budgets.

Don't put yourself last.

Note: these lists are intended to inspire you, not restrict you. None of this is fully comprehensive. Toss out ideas and keep what you like! Have fun, and we'll see you at the end of the aisle.

Keep in mind your guests' needs while looking at venues, not just your own. The following requirements may also be good reminders for your benchmarks.

Easily accessible bathrooms

Plenty of individual toilets

Wheelchair access

Smooth terrain

Ample parking

Enough seating for your guest list

Let's begin with something of a catch-all: chronic pain. If you have chronic pain, you tire easily. And get sore. And cranky. You'll need your royal tower (not literally … no stairs here!) to hide out in should *you* become the dragon. This list is not meant to be exhaustive; however, it is intended to be used as a useful inspirational tool for those whose conditions cause chronic pain.

A nice house venue is a great option for relaxed people with chronic pain. These you can rent out for the weekend and house out-of-town guests in, or you could find a friend or family member who could let you use the house for the day for free. Designate a room as the wedding suite, have your ceremony and reception at the house, and retreat whenever you need a break.

If you want something more chic, try a hotel. The more upscale version of the house venue, many hotels come with wedding planners built in and a restaurant that caters to all diets. You'll still have your wedding suite to retreat to, and an upside: wheelchair ramps and elevators!

For elegant sophistication, try a historic mansion. Many state capitols have these, as well as old, historic cities. Sometimes you'll find these out in the countryside in the middle of nowhere. Occasionally, these have all-inclusive wedding packages.

Religious venues can also be good choices for those with chronic pain. Fred and Rachel were married in their local church in the village where they had both lived their entire lives after Fred graduated university. The only other venue was a half hour away, and with Rachel's chronic pain, this was not possible. Their reception was in the function room of a castle nearby. Fred and Rachel live in Scotland.

Meagan, who has a rare, life-threatening, painful disease, chose a cheap chapel built by German prisoners of war (POWs) with an all-inclusive wedding package. Another reason why she chose the venue was because the venue was beautiful, and she did not have to waste time and money decorating it herself. The venue was found on a ghost tour. She planned ahead for her symptoms by working with her doctor for a plan for her wedding day. Think outside the box and anything can be yours.

Speaking of thinking outside the box, all aboard! Time for a destination cruise wedding. You'll get a 3-in-1! Wedding, reception, and a honeymoon. These are usually small, intimate ceremonies that don't last long, and are typically referred to as "Weddingmoons." You'll have your honeymoon suite to retreat to whenever you like, and food galore!

Many mobility aid users also suffer from chronic pain, so there will be some overlap here. Mobility aids range from a cane to a power wheelchair, and anything else that helps you move. It's important that you can move at your venue – but remember that these are suggestions. Look for what inspires you in the real world. If you fall in love with a place that isn't 100% accessible, try asking for an accommodation. Most places are happy to help. If they aren't, move on. The perfect one will come along.

Let's start with the obvious: hotels. These are very mobility-aid friendly with ramps and elevators, and usually quite elegant. You can choose your wedding suite to be disability-friendly. Hotels offering wedding services almost always come with a full wedding crew.

Hotels make excellent choices for wheelchair users. Oftentimes, they are the premiere local venue. These venues can require less travel, a bonus for mobility aid users. Carrie-Ann, who uses a wheelchair, says "Our venue was the Grange Hotel. It was the only actual venue that we physically visited, though we discounted a lot of others looking at bro- chures, etc. It was important to me that we could have the ceremony and reception at one venue. Wheelchair access was paramount. We wanted somewhere close to where we live, meaning that we didn't want to be tied into taking a certain number of the hotel's bedrooms. Cost was an important factor as we weren't on a huge budget." Narrowing her search through distance, Carrie-Ann settled on the hotel without having to travel much to find a venue during the wedding planning process.

Due to travel and accessibility, urban locations are good for mobility, so our next stop is the public library. These are most likely located in a city center and fitted for wheelchair access through the front door for a proper wedding entrance. The library should be up to date on city building code. Some libraries have very beautiful and charming architecture. If you're a bibliophile, this is your place.

Another urban location is a modern chapel at a state university. Think a younger state school with an all-faiths chapel. Older chapels may have uneven stone surfaces. If you can't check this out in person, have someone in your wedding party – or your wedding planner – do a virtual tour. But be sure that it's modern and fitted to your needs: ramp, bathroom stalls, door opening devices, and smooth surfaces to move on. It's best if you can check these out yourself.

Further in our urban adventure is an art gallery in town. Fun for artsy folks, these are usually near a downtown epicenter, and fitted for access through the front door. The novelty of it will woo your guests, as will the ambiance from the one-of-a-kind artwork.

An alternative for the cultured couple in an urban setting is a museum, also typically fitted for mobility with beautiful architecture and features. These can be as intellectual or as whimsical as you want – if you have children, want a kid-friendly wedding, or are simply children at heart, consider a children's museum.

Now let's head out of the city and into the woods to a destination wedding for some ideas for those with rustic tastes. Hear me out on this one, but some national parks in the United States are very upscale and fully fit for wheelchairs, canes and walkers. These include the Grand Canyon, which I recommend most for accessibility. They have officiants, five-star restaurants and luxury hotels. Most have fully paved walkways and resemble theme parks more than deserted forests. Next stop on our destination journey is Disneyworld! Disney offers all-inclusive packages starting at $5,000 that includes a reception meal and a wedding planner, among other things. Just show up with your dress. Disney is known for its accessibility. If you are a fan, why not?

Tips for Finding Your True Venue

If you have mobility problems, it may take you longer to find a venue with accessibility suitable for a wedding. Allow for two-to-four times longer in your wedding planning schedule to find a wedding venue. Don't worry, the perfect venue will come along!

Here are some tips to finding your true venue in a timely manner:

Look online first. Meagan looked at 50 venues online before only looking at two in person – her ceremony site and reception venue. When you go to see a venue, or Skype someone going to a potential venue, make a list of your symptoms and how certain things in the environment you live in irritate you. Bring the list with you and read it aloud, scoping it out for pitfalls. Make a Google Spreadsheet (sheets.google.com or the Google Sheets app in the Google Play Store or App store for iOS) of each venue with a row for each question (such as 1, 2, 3...) and put an X by each one that fails. The venue with the least number of Xs wins your wedding venue.

A Tale of Two Venues

I planned two weddings, and therefore had two venues. Both were reception and ceremony ready. In this book I've already talked about my parents' Victorian fairytale, which was my second venue. My first venue was a children's camp a family friend of ours managed.

Multiple weddings had been thrown there. Most weddings I had ever been to took place at the camp. It was beautiful: picturesque with waterfalls, cliffs, and green rolling hills. I knew it was what my husband and I could afford and that he would love it.

We had a down payment of $60 for 24 hours and a special of $600 for the discounted venue. It was typically $1000. We received this discount because of the 15 year long friendship I had with the camp manager's family. My husband, a botanist and avid outdoorsman, loved it. Not to mention on the highest cliff in the camp stood three white crosses overlooking the creek we chose our ceremony site to be next to.

But with my illness, I was transforming. Little by little I was fading away. The girl who spent hours outside on the trail after work was diminishing. I was no longer rugged and mucky. As much as I could appreciate plants and animals, I couldn't drive all the way to the camp, cross a bridge by foot twice, and have a wedding.

Besides, feral hogs had previously torn up the ceremony site, leaving grown-over holes in the ground, and I was wearing kitten heels. What if I caught my foot and fell?

Needless to say, the camp couldn't accommodate me and it wasn't "me." It was beautiful, but it didn't suit my vibe.

I had booked the camp before my mobility issues appeared. No one can predict the future, and I have the more important ring on my finger anyway.

This is to say, take heart in your wedding planning – no matter what unforeseen circumstances arise, know that you are loved. You deserve that love, and you deserve the best venue.

Photography

Book your photographer as soon as you have your venue, which should pretty much be as soon as you are engaged. Photographers book up fast, so be quick, but read reviews and check out their portfolios!

Consider hiring a newbie, someone with a side business, or an amateur, as long as you have seen their portfolios and approve. A college student is also a good choice. The general rule of thumb is "Do I like their work? Do they photograph people like me?" If you're iffy, it's also okay to email, text, or call to ask questions. Many photographers have hidden photoshoots they may share when asked. Questions to consider include what your venue's lighting is, such as whether or not it is indoors or outdoors, yellow or blue light, if they have photographed at certain times of day and what types of weather conditions, when contacting a photographer about examples of their work.

Disclose, Disclose, Disclose!

The number one rule with all vendors is to disclose all the nitty gritty of your disability during the hiring process. I found that because I had explained my conditions to my vendors, I was able to change the dates due to my medical emergency. That was huge!

One of the things my photographer did was have me stay seated during bridal portraits and keep me off my feet as much as possible during my wedding. I was having trouble walking and disclosed to her throughout my engagement all the crazy medical mumbo-jumbo that was going on. She understood perfectly and never took pictures of me in pain.

Something that I noticed about my photographer was that she asked me who my partner was when she met me – this is a good sign for LGBTQ+ soonlyweds. When scoping out your photographer, pay attention to their website – can you sense their beliefs? What do they value? Who do they usually shoot? Is who they photograph similar to how you look or want to look on your big day? Next, ensure the use of appropriate pronouns.

Videographers

Affordable videographers can be found on Thumbtack, and consider hiring local off of Facebook for deals if you're getting married in your area. If not, the Knot and WeddingWire have plenty of professionals to choose from. A way to save money is to have the videographer mic your officiant, music, and the couple and shoot raw footage. The videographer will give the raw footage to someone the couple knows, and they will edit the footage as a wedding gift. Or, if you know someone good with cameras, they can shoot and edit video for you. Just be sure to have mics for everyone involved in the ceremony and whatever parts of the reception you want.

Flowers

Flowers are another crucial part of your vision that tie in with décor. Should you have them at all? Or should you have them somewhat, or in droves?

There's another dimension to flowers … sensory or non-sensory. Are flowers part of your sensory problems? Do their fragrances give you migraines?

If you have people writing in on your RSVP cards with sensitivities to smells, or you have flower allergies, you might not want real flowers. That's okay! That doesn't mean you have to DIY from Hobby Lobby. Most traditional, stand-alone florists will still make silk arrangements for you. They can also remove the stamens from real flowers to cut down on smells and allergens so you can still have them.

On the other hand, if flowers are one of your favorite things, you are highly sensory and like to associate happy memories with smells, I've got a show stopper for you: grocery store florists.

These are not the flowers next to the check-out. Most grocery stores in the United States and Canada have a florist working on site, and you can ask them to do your wedding flowers. Common grocery stores with florists include Tesco and Costco.

Bouquets, like the rest of your flowers, are perfectly fine things to get from a grocery florist. However, if you need accommodations, you might want to go to a traditional florist. For example, a wheelchair user had a wrist corsage instead of a traditional bouquet so they could push themselves down the aisle. The corsage served as their wedding ceremony flowers. Another reason to use a traditional florist for special circumstances is if you use a walker or cane. If you do, they can be decorated by your florist to act as a bouquet and be part of your special day.

It's best to contact a florist 12-6 months out from your wedding day, as florists book up fast the way photographers do. This is especially true if you are tying the knot during peak wedding season. Peak wedding season varies where you live, but for most parts of the northern hemisphere it is May through the end of June.

If you have a 12-month engagement, send your floral designs to your florist 6-4 months out. You can find inspiration on Pinterest or even in nature. Florists can also help you create designs based on your colors and seasonal flowers. If your wedding is 6 months out, the rule is 6-4 months out for a design.

When confirming a floral order, have your wedding planner, day-of coordinator, or yourself call the florist 2-3 days in advance to ensure everything is good to go. You'll learn who is picking up the flowers when and where.

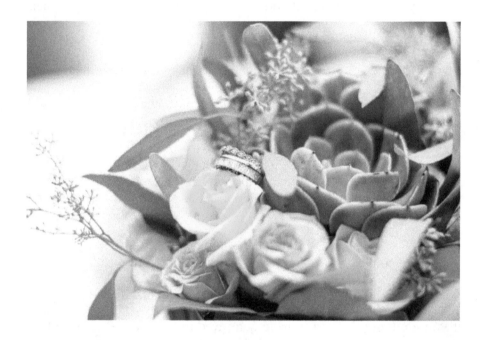

Image Credit: Tauni Joy Photography

My Texas-Style grocery florist bridal bouquet consisting of green succulents, light pink small roses, yellow roses, eucalyptus, and baby's breath. The bouquet has much greenery to save money. In the middle of the bouquet are my husband and my wedding rings – a gray sparkling meteorite men's band and a rose gold diamond baguette women's wedding band on top of the men's band.

Invitations

Your invitations should fit your vision, or theme of the wedding. Try to incorporate your wedding colors into the invitation so your guests know what they are.

Basic Guidelines

Generally speaking, if you have a six-month engagement, save the dates go out one month after you get engaged. Invitations go out two months before the wedding. If you have a year before the wedding, save the dates go out six months before the wedding, and invitations out two months before your special date.

However, for the sake of having a disability-friendly wedding, send the invitations out once you have a venue. This does break decorum, but for your own comfort during the planning process and your guests at the wedding, it's good to keep in mind others' needs, which you will use your RSVP cards to collect.

Writing Invitations

Save the dates aren't very important. They should be a cute memento that you exist, and "Hey! We're getting married on this date, put this on your calendar, expect something from us later." Save the dates are completely optional, and do not have to be sent if you don't want to. They also serve as a way to announce your engagement.

Invitations... polite wars have been fought over invitations.

Invitations come in two parts, the front pretty invitation, and the RSVP Card, which is arguably more important.

Note: Double-check your send-by date.

The Basic Special Accommodations RSVP Card Template

X_____

Person's Name Here

RSVP? YES NO

PLUS __

Do you have the following sensitivities:

Food   Sensory   Drink   Mobility

Write details on back and send by XX/XX/XXXX

Wedding Websites

Wedding websites are a far more popular alternative to paper invitations. Many may still send them out for posterity's sake, but websites such as weddingwire.com or theknot.com have virtual RSVPs and invitations. This means they can be screen-read. Websites created on Wedding Wire are free to create and will be easier on your pocketbook should you decide to go paperless.

You can recreate the Basic Special Accommodations RSVP Card Template on your wedding website for people to fill out when they RSVP. Their data will be easier to keep up with.

A note on wedding registries: as someone who is disabled, you may be loath to go out to a store and pick out your wedding gifts. You can now do wedding registries completely online and share them on your wedding website. Or you can opt not to do them at all!

Your Nearest and Dearest: the Wedding Party

Planning a wedding comes with fun and interesting challenges. You're only going to want the people who love you most and are the most reliable in your circle on your team.

It's suggested to have larger wedding parties when you are disabled so you have more attendees should something go wrong wedding-wise or health wise. The wedding party is like your little cloud of worker bees – they're there to help you throughout the process, and ultimately on your special day.

When deciding who to choose to be in your wedding party, ask yourself:

Who always answers my phone calls, even if it's after dark?

Who always texts me back?

Who has consistently been there for me when I needed it most?

Your wedding party is supposed to be there to watch out for you, and in a disability case, keep guard. Rachel looks back on her wedding now that Fred has epilepsy and wishes that he would have "people whose job it was to keep an eye on him, someone knowing where he is all the time, bring him drinks etc. Probably several people, and not parents as they would have their own guests to greet etc. Likely his sister, or best man. Just that extra support so that he doesn't end up having a seizure somewhere without someone noticing." The wedding party has a job whether or not the couple is disabled. They are almost like a security team for the couple.

The point is, you need reliable, dependable people on your team. Remember that your true friends can know you for a year or ten years; the length of the friendship doesn't dictate the quality. Second point: you don't have to have the same number on your side as your partner's. Third point: don't feel pressured to have your partner's family, or your family, be in your wedding party! Fourthly, you don't have to restrict your side of the wedding party to your gender. An example would be K. W. Warburton's wedding party, who "had 3 bridesmaids and 1 brides-man. My husband had 3 groomsmen." Don't forget your folx wedding attendants, to be covered in the Clothes section of the book.

Dangers of Matching With Your Partner

As I've said before, we had a house wedding with 20 guests. But we didn't have hired help, which meant my little family was running around doing everything – from making the music work, serving food, to ensuring the pets weren't let out.

An easy way to ensure that we could have had help without hiring someone was that I decided not to match my partner with my side of the wedding party. He only had one person, and I had several female friends I grew up with who said we would be each other's bridesmaids or maids of honor. I decided not to embarrass him and only choose my sister as my maid of honor.

My house wedding was not a disaster, but I feel for my family for working so hard and not enjoying the night. They needed an extra pair of hands.

Hotel Blocks

Let's arrange a hotel room for each guest. We'll go step-by-step.

Step #1. For out-of-town guests, you'll want to find hotels that give "courtesy blocks" – blocks of rooms where you don't have to pay for any unsold rooms. A quick way to find these is HiSkipper.com.

Step #2. Be sure to call the hotel to make sure the hotel you're selecting is, in fact, offering courtesy blocks.

Step #3. Ask the hotel questions to determine Step #2

How many rooms do you need to reserve before you can fill a block?

If you don't fill a room, are there any penalties?

What is the room rate?

Will the rooms in the block be close together?

Can we add more rooms? Is there an extra fee?

What is included with the block?

Is this hotel close to an airport? Is there a shuttle or any other transportation?

Step #4. Once you've found your courtesy block at your hotel, the hotel will email the info to you, and you can put the info on your wedding website or forward the email.

Wedding Planners & Others

If thrifty DIY isn't your thing, go to your local bridal expo and look for a highly rated day-of coordinator. Not everyone needs a wedding planner, but pretty much all weddings need a day-of coordinator. If you believe you need a wedding planner, and many of you may feel this as well, go to your local bridal expo and find that highly experienced wedding planner and give them their chance to shine. Ask the wedding planners you encounter questions about your disability to determine if they're a good fit. See if your partner or a member of the wedding party can video chat you at the bridal expo because they are huge all-day events if you can't get out that day. If you decide to disclose your condition to your wedding planner, do so immediately while hiring them instead of later. K. W. Warburton, who has postural orthostatic tachycardia syndrome (POTS) told me, "Everything was going smoothly until I disclosed my illness and requirements to the wedding planner 2 months before my big day. Communications were sporadic after that and they didn't even show up on the actual day! My maid of honor even had to take over and organize the cake." It's safe to say to always, absolutely disclose as soon as you can to everyone in your wedding crew!

Of course, some venues come with wedding planners, like K. W. Warburton's. Disclose to your venue and staff upon hiring. If you're reading this wondering when to hire a wedding planner, it should be in the two months after you get engaged, or simply when you feel like you're drowning. The best wedding planners are flexible and can whip up a wedding in a month.

When do you know you need a wedding planner? If you or your partner has a demanding job, either of you lives away from your parents, or you have a destination wedding. Difficult family dynamics, either partners having severe anxiety, and large weddings usually require a full-service wedding planner. Some wedding planners focus on one particular specialty – such as wedding invitation design – but many are full-service, especially in this day and age.

The previously mentioned day-of coordinator can be less expensive but very supportive, depending on who you hire. They are great for smaller weddings. Typically you have two meetings with them before the wedding and have email support for questions, and they work with you on Google Docs for a timeline, playlist, and vendor contact information directory, depending on how tech-savvy both of you are. It is important to mention that day-of coordinators also work the rehearsal dinner. Depending on how your contract, they can help serve food and might have a food license. The day-of coordinator will also set up your ceremony and reception décor.

Wedding Clothes

The Shoes

The shoes are more important than the dress. Yes, I said it. Why?

Because if you have comfy shoes, you will be happier throughout the day. If you have uncomfortable shoes, you will be upset all day. You'll feel your feet burning even while sitting down.

What are the world's comfiest wedding shoes?

I'm glad you asked!

You won't like this first one. I know Crocs are associated with dads, high socks, and tourists, but hear me out … Crocs makes Crocs that don't look like Crocs. They make dress Crocs that look like ballet flats and sandals. Honestly, they're cute.

I had bought some before my wedding in desperation for a summer shoe. But the idea of the Crocs stigma lingering over my bridal essence scared me.

So, I went out in kitten heels. Do not go out in kitten heels! Not even those! If you must wear kitten heels, or heels at all, there is a tactic to wearing them. "I wore kitten heels for the ceremony, because heels make my joint pain worse. When we arrived at the reception venue, I changed into trainers. They were new but well-worn in inside the house" – Rachel had a similar experience to mine, but she planned ahead by breaking in her sneakers.

After the ceremony I was in so much pain from my kitten heels. I went to my room to lay down, and my husband took my beautiful but traitorous kitten heels off my feet. We found my white Crocs sandals and I slipped them on. I was 110% better.

Storytelling aside, the most comfortable dress shoes are white dress Crocs, Dr. Scholl's Ballet flats, and Converse All Stars.

Wedding Attire

When you were little, how did you imagine yourself when you dreamed? Were you in a fairytale in a glittery ballgown? A warrior? A powerful queen? Or were you like me – you wanted to be a dragon?

Answering these questions will lead you to what your wedding clothes vision is. Your wedding clothes vision is more important than your ability. As you read through the following sections, hold on to this fallen star and remember to make your dreams come true no matter the odds.

Wedding Dresses

If you suffer from chronic pain, the dress will be a big factor in how your wedding day will go. This is because it dictates your comfort level. There are easy ways to figure this out without wasting energy trying on tons of dresses, which will drain your energy.

Chronic pain spans over many abilities listed in this book, so if you think this applies to you, feel free to take notes.

Tips for figuring out which dresses to try on

Consider a non-bridal dress that happens to be white. These will have fewer layers and will be less heavy, and less expensive. I try to be budget-friendly in this book because I know with medical expenses, everything else can get in the way. It's best to prioritize your health.

Rachel's dress was "a custom-made long princess-cut ballgown with a corset underneath, which was really hot, as our wedding day ended up being the warmest day of the year." Keep in mind what season your wedding is in when considering what kind of dress you want. "I had a detachable train, as I didn't want the extra weight as I was scared of falling or tripping, which I did a lot as I got tired. I had a veil but it didn't ever go over my face, it was always positioned at the back of my head." This was for mobility purposes, which is part of why exhaustion and big dresses can be pretty but also a problem for brides with chronic pain.

A way to do this is to look for a dress with only two or three layers. Wedding dresses are like cakes. Some have more fabric layers than most. Some have up to 12, and this makes the dress heavy. The heavier the dress, the more uncomfortable you will feel as it places pressure on your body, causing pain and exhaustion.

A way to calculate the pain level of a dress is its fabric. The softer and lighter it is, the better. Jersey knit, lace and satin are gentle on the skin.

Make sure you bring a flashlight to test if the fabric is see-through!

It's common for those with chronic pain to have body fluctuations. This can be due to their illness, an injury, or a number of factors. If your weight fluctuates, consider a corset top. Try a soft corset top that will lace-up all the way with a ribbon. That means that no matter how your body changes, the dress can be altered through tightening or loosening the corset lacing. Be sure that if you buy a corset lace-up top that it is soft and has no hard boning structure that can be felt.

Where Should You Buy a Dress?

Most lightweight dresses are not found in traditional bridal shops, so I suggest getting creative with your search. One idea is shopping at a secondhand bridal shop. This way, you can buy couture for less, and get it off the rack the same day. Another idea is Quinceañera shops. There you can find excellent customer service and a different style of dress if you don't like current bridal fashion. Department stores are wonderful places to find dresses with fewer layers. The dresses will be simpler and more low-key, and a simpler dress is usually a more comfortable dress. The best department stores to find a wedding dress are Nordstrom and Macy's.

How to Shop

In order to see how comfortable the dress is on your body, try not to shop online. Only go to one store per day. When you dress shop, make it your one goal for the day. Or if you need to shop online, try a mail-in wedding dress subscription service and try on one dress per day, as these will be traditional wedding dresses and hefty. Mail-in wedding dress subscription services send you three designer grade dresses in the mail at a time. Try them on and send back what you don't like, and only pay for the one (or two) dresses you truly love.

Shapewear

Try to wear as little shapewear and other undergarments as possible. This means no complicated slips or spandex. You're going to need to pee at some point. These items are also restrictive and uncomfortable. If you do wear spandex, make sure they are soft to the touch, almost velveteen, and flexible. Additionally, invest in a high-quality comfortable strapless bra.

Focus on Your Physical Pain Areas

If you have abdominal pain from endometriosis or a spasming gallbladder, an empire waist dress might be in order, as the dress will flow over your abdomen and not touch you at all. Consider the softness of the fabric and a beachy halter top or an elegant drop waist to keep the pressure off of your ribcage if you have pain there.

Focus on your painful areas and make sure the dress doesn't cling to them. You will be beautiful in any dress, but will you be comfortable in each of them?

Comfort should be a big factor for anyone looking for a wedding dress, not just those with chronic pain, but we all have different values. Those with mobility aids may have chronic pain and find this information useful for their wedding dress shopping. Even if they don't, comfort and ease of wear are typically factors for mobility aid users, especially wheelchair users.

Many different kinds of people use wheelchairs. The types of wheelchair users discussed in this chapter are not exhaustive. Please note that with finding the right dress, and sometimes altering it appropriately, any wheelchair user can wear any dress. Here are some suggestions from real wheelchair users to provide inspiration, not limitations.

Comfort and style were two big factors for Carrie-Ann in her search for the dress of her dreams. Carrie-Ann, who has cerebral palsy, told me, "The dress that I wanted didn't exist in bridal shops – it was almost the top of one dress, and the skirt of another. So that's exactly what I went with, a two-piece corset and long skirt, custom-made by Bridal Dream Dress. This was a style preference, but it also made sitting in my wheelchair more comfortable with more flexibility on the waist." Top and bottom separates can also be found in stores. These are also good choices for paraplegics for mobility purposes, as a potential choice.

A dress doesn't have to be custom-made or need many alterations to be a good choice for a wheelchair user. You might find something right off the rack that needs minimal alterations, such as hemming.

Sometimes wheelchair users gravitate toward certain types of dresses due to mobility. It's common for motorized wheelchair users to wear short or tea-length wedding dresses. Those looking for a pop of color or more personality might sew a colorful petticoat into a tea-length dress so guests will have something interesting to look at while they are seated.

You can also dress up your chair! Drape it with lace or white satin and flowers. Let everyone know that all parts of you are special, beautiful, and to be celebrated.

Or, you could have a wedding chair. Carrie-Ann did not use her daily use wheelchair and instead bought an antique one. She spray-painted it white and decorated it with fabric. Carrie-Ann also urges all disabled people to not rule any dress out just because they use a wheelchair.

A Tale of Two Dresses

You know how it's trendy to have a reception dress and a wedding dress, and this is how girls end up with two dresses? Yeah, no. This is not that story.

My mama raised me to think that girls who had multiple wedding dresses were selfish and wasteful. (Besides, in debt.) After all, I only spent $199 on my first dress. Imagine my embarrassment when I found myself in a two-dress predicament.

My two-dress predicament began with medication. I was swollen up like a balloon. The cute, soft, lacey little sheath wedding dress I had bought the week of my engagement – which was a mistake – was too form-fitting and I cried every time I looked at myself in it. When I wore it I could barely sit in it.

First of all, when I watched an episode of Say Yes to the Dress, I realized a plain lace sheath was not what I wanted. When Randy pulled out that Lazaro sparkle-all-over ballgown, I dreamed in glitter henceforth. I even called secondhand stores about the dress. It was thousands of dollars out of my price range.

Then, someone I considered to be a good friend came over to my house and saw my photo I kept by my computer monitor of me in the dress as inspiration and trashed it. Thoroughly. She was even there when I picked out the dress!

I cried after she left and immediately sought places to buy a wedding dress for $200 or less. That was all the money I honestly had. After calling around and getting the rude response or two of "If you're honestly going to spend *that* little on a wedding dress ..." I found a Quinceañera shop who could accommodate me.

Let me tell you, they had the best dresses out of any I had seen at any bridal store. It was like a time warp back to the 90s, and I was all about that. I discussed with the retail clerk my health problems, and the perfect dress came to me.

It was a simple, elegant, empire waist princess dress with glittery sequins on the bodice. It fit perfectly. My mother smiled, the first dress she'd ever smiled at – she hadn't even smiled at the first one I bought.

This dress was a sparkly princess dress, and I was a fairytale princess in my wedding vision. It even twirled, something a sheath couldn't do, and above all, the glitter on the bodice made me shine.

Did I cry? No. But was I blissfully happy? Yes.

Dressing the Wedding Party

Dressing your wedding party comes down to preference, but not just yours. Your wedding attendants will have needs, such as budget and body type comfort. Some may want to show up in jeans and cowboy hats. It's easy to get angry at this part, but for the sake of your friendships, please don't.

Attendant Dresses

Remember your vision. Do you have a romantic theme in mind, or something more sleek and modern? Are you relaxed and comfortable or classic? If you want, call in to mind the texture of your dress and the fabric. Attendant dresses can be found at any department store as a more affordable alternative to a bridal shop. A favorite is JC Penney for its cute dresses and low prices.

Many bridal stores will match your wedding colors and fabric swatches for your attendant dresses. Simply come into the store and an attendant will match for you. A good brick-and-mortar example of this is David's Bridal. There are also many online retailers who do this and specialize in wedding attendants.

Suits

The most important thing about the suits is that they coordinate, they go with your vision, and you're happy with them. For a classic tux, try Men's Warehouse for rentals. They partner with David's Bridal for deals. Or, consider keeping it in the family for sentimentality and budget. My partner wore my grandfather's seersucker suit tailored to fit him. His best man wore his favorite suit. If you're having a casual wedding, ask your partner what they like to wear to feel attractive. For some, this is dark-wash Wrangler jeans and cowboy boots! As long as you're happy, though, it's okay.

If someone in your wedding party is disabled and requires dress pants, there are a few options. A wheelchair user should use Gabardine dress pants. The Tommy Hilfiger Adaptive brand available at Macy's includes formal pants. Kohl's also has the MagnaClick line of formal pants good for a wheelchair user. Any type of pants that are specifically made to make it easier to get them on and off are great pants to have for your partner.

For wheelchair users needing a dress jacket, have a tailor make a short jacket that would come halfway down their torso on a standing person. This cropped jacket would hit a person sitting in a chair right at the waist and not get tangled in anyone's wheels. The illusion is the same as a full-length dress jacket on someone who is standing.

For partners with chronic pain, please let them have a bit more say in what they wear. If you're having a July wedding and they are in a wool suit with a scratchy shirt, reconsider. You want them to enjoy the wedding, too. Fabrics cause pain in those with chronic pain, and those who identify as somewhere else on the gender spectrum than you are no different.

Male sufferers of chronic pain do exist, and should be accommodated. When I asked Stephen, who has fibromyalgia which causes chronic pain, if he had any accommodations made to his attire, he told me he wore "a suit. No modification. But wish I had asked for a fan! The church was really warm as we started." Stephen suffers from overheating, so this was a big problem. Perhaps be creative when dressing your partner, or brainstorm ways to accommodate them, such as a decorative paper fan in Stephen's case.

At the time Fred and Rachel were married, Fred did not yet have epilepsy. Looking back, Rachel would change a few things about Fred's attire, as they were married in the summer. He "wore a full kilt, which looked incredible, but is all wool and is extremely hot. If our wedding was now, he would still want a kilt but we would picked a different date to stop him from overheating. He would also now change into his own shoes after the ceremony, as he can be unstable on his feet and the kilt shoes don't offer much grip." If Fred had epilepsy when they got married, these would be the attire accommodations Rachel would make for him now. Like Rachel, please keep in mind your partner.

Flower Girl, Ring Bearer, and Pets

Many bridal stores and salons, including David's Bridal, have full flower girl and ring bearer pairings to purchase with your dress. Consider purchasing your flower girl and ring bearer clothes when deciding on your dress to have assistance from staff and your entourage. Amazon.com is also a great place to find ring bearer and flower girl accessories and attire for a more affordable price.

For those of you who don't have any young children in your family circles, consider a flower dog, ring dog, dog of honor or best dog! Costumes for dogs can be found at David's Bridal, major pet retailers, and Amazon.com. As my husband and I did not have young nieces, nephews, or cousins, we opted for a flower dog.

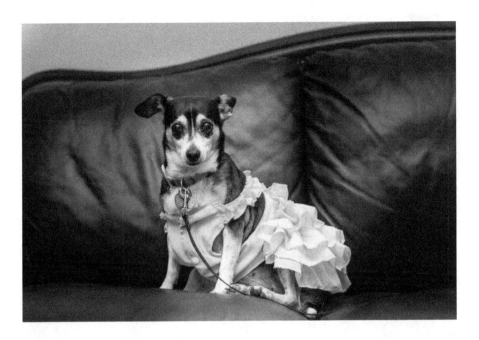

Photo Credit: Tauni Joy Photography

Small dog with black, tan, and white fur with pointed ears and a delicate muzzle in a pink ruffled dress on a brown leather couch.

Refreshments

Caterer and Baker

Allergies and special diets are rife within our world today, not just the disabled community. But many disabled people have special diets that could mean the difference between a good and bad day, as do their families and friends.

I recommend the Thumbtack app for finding a good, low-cost, quality baker who can accommodate multiple food allergies and dietary needs for your wedding cake. In the Thumbtack app, there is a useful virtual form that lets you input allergies when you contact a caterer or baker. They will decide if and how to respond to you.

There are certain types of cuisine more likely to hit across the board for food sensitivities. A couple that come to mind are Mediterranean and Italian. Shopping local for your mom and pop restaurant is another good way to get a good deal. If you know of a good local restaurant, first try them before going to Thumbtack, such as your local mom and pop Italian restaurant or gyro eatery.

When you sent out your RSVP cards or collected info on your wedding website, you should have figured out the general food sensitivities and diets of your guests. When it comes to caterers, there's no need to book them months out. Contact your caterer at least two weeks before your big day to work out the details of your menu with you and your guests' dietary needs in mind.

Alternatives to Catering Traditional Style

While I did have catering at my wedding, it was done buffet-style with friends serving to save money. I had a local mom and pop Italian restaurant drop off one enormous pan of food that served 25 people. You could also have your friends help in other ways, such as putting on a potluck or barbecue. Also, you do not have to serve meals at weddings. Consider a dessert buffet with snack food trays from large grocery stores like Costco and baked goods from a local bakery tailored to everyone's dietary needs.

Drinks

Even if you want to have an open bar, it's important to remember all of your guests. Not everyone at your wedding will want or be able to drink. It's also common sense to have plenty of water. Have cisterns of water and non-alcoholic alternatives for those who don't drink alcohol. You might fall into that category. Says K. W. Warburton, "Because of my POTS, I am not able to drink alcohol so I arranged for a non-alcoholic alternative for myself. Unfortunately, I was still given a glass of champagne when I arrived. I can't manage large meals, so we chose to have an afternoon tea style wedding reception instead of the standard 3-course meal so that I could enjoy the food without fear of overloading my stomach." You can ensure everyone, including yourself, is accommodated. Even if something goes wrong, you can still enjoy a tea-time reception.

Music

Music adds to the ambiance of the wedding. It's an expression of your tastes and what you value. Some of you may love music, others of you may only listen to the Top 40 and not pay much more attention to it. That's fine. There is no correct or incorrect way to have music at your wedding.

You can have music that matches your theme. If you want a more fuss-free, down-to earth wedding, consider hiring someone with an acoustic guitar. This could even be a friend or a college student if you want to be budget-friendly. Or, if you are having a more highbrow wedding, hire classical music students from a local university, such as a cellist or a string quartet, to complement your black tie theme. Then, of course, you have your rock and roll weddings – you can find listings of wedding bands online, or if you're in a band, you probably know of some already.

Many weddings opt for DJs due to ease and versatility of genre. With a DJ, you can skip from country to R&B in minutes with your own curated playlist you give to the DJ. If you should want one, find and book a DJ four months out. DJs can sometimes be booked last minute, depending on how popular your wedding date is.

But if you have problems with migraines and want a DJ, can you still have one? Yes!

Let's go over the steps for arranging accommodations with your DJ.

If you have sensory problems that give you pain and migraines, disclose to the DJ your sensory problems and give them explicit directions on what they can and cannot do during the hiring process. Directions include whether or not lights can be brought, what kind of lights, if fog machines can be brought, and the volume level of the music. If they say they can't do it, don't hire. If they can, great. This all can make your DJ price cheaper, too, by cutting down on accessories.

The most cheap and laid-back end of this is the iPod DJ, where you designate a friend or family member to play music from your passcode-locked iPod for the remainder of the wedding. Just make sure the iPod is always in a safe family member or friend's hands the entire wedding, and is never left alone.

Sound Systems

If your wedding is outdoors or you have a group above fifty in attendance, you're going to need to rent a sound system. Even if you have someone playing an acoustic guitar, they will need to be mic'd if you're outdoors and there's a highway behind you. You can find good rates on sound equipment from local music stores. They can even set it all up for you for a small extra fee. Sound systems can be rented one to two weeks out from the wedding from your local music store.

A DJ can set up a sound system for you as well with their equipment if the reception and ceremony are in the same place, or both locations should they be in different areas if they are part of an audio-visual company. You can find DJs at bridal expos or on the Thumbtack app, as well as recommendations from your other vendors. A DJ should be hired at the same time as your other musicians would be.

Your Music Does Not Have to Match the Venue

My husband and I are both into jazz. We like to swing dance and have friends who do as well. When we had our rustic venue, we didn't plan on playing country music. It was all big band, jazz and swing as if we were dancing out of a black and white film … into a honky-tonk in the woods. Which might not make sense to some people. So no, your music does not have to match the venue, but if you have a theme, it helps if it does. We were serving Italian food and playing Frank Sinatra, so for us it made some sense.

Cosmetologists

As most people prefer a fresh, basic look for their wedding day, many cosmetologists can do this with ease with little time. However, they are costly, usually in the $150 range minimum for makeup alone. Hair usually costs the same, for about $300 combined. Going to a makeup store like Ulta or Sephora can save you cash on a fresh face, and having your beauty-savvy friend is even more pocket-friendly. However, use caution at Ulta or Sephora as many of the makeup artists there are rookies. Communicate with your makeup artist thoroughly, whether they are seasoned or a newbie.

It is best to book your cosmetologist six months to a year in advance from your wedding, as they do book up quickly.

Transportation

For the Couple

Pamper yourself on your wedding day! Instead of driving yourself around, make your cosmetologists come to you. Have your wedding attendants drive you to the venue and beauty appointments. Or, the more fun options would be hiring a car and chauffeur or a limo: get yourself and your wedding party to the venue in style!

There is another option to get to the venue, taken from Carrie-Ann: "I decided to stay at the venue the night before the wedding and get ready there, to lessen stress and time pressure in the morning. We arranged a coach to transport guests to and from the wedding." This is a bonus for staying at a hotel or house venue.

You can arrange for transportation during the month of your wedding, should you choose to hire it. Two to three days before, call to confirm with your driver how to get to the airport for your honeymoon.

For Your Guests

There's a few things you could do here, especially if you're having alcohol served at your wedding.

First, it might be unwise to have your wedding somewhere remote. This is because remote locations do not have rideshares, and chauffeured transportation will be extremely expensive.
If you are somewhere where there are rideshares, assign someone in your wedding party to order rides for your guests.

For a more luxurious trip for your guests, hire a party shuttle to bring your guests to and from their hotel. Lastly, consider a house wedding. Have all your guests stay at the house, and no one will need rides. Likewise, having a hotel wedding and reception venue will solve this problem.

Rentals

Rentals can be found at your venue, sometimes at no extra cost. Other times, these connections can be found at your bridal expo. What's important is negotiating a contract – how long will you have the rentals, what condition do you need to return them in, and when do you need to return them? You may have someone in the wedding party return the rentals for you if you're leaving for your honeymoon the day after. If not, you could return them yourself the day after or the week after, whenever the contract dictates.

You can rent almost anything, from different types of décor to tents, dance floors, table settings, linens, to chairs and archways. Rentals may or may not be cheaper depending on your area or whether or not you have a savvy wedding planner or day-of coordinator with connections. A bonus to having these types of wedding professionals is that they can usually bargain deals for you and arrange everything for you in advance so you don't have to worry.

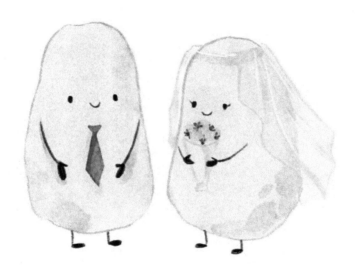

The Extras

Items in this section are still important to the ambiance of your wedding, but don't involve vendors so much as the previous section.

Decor

There are many ways to handle décor. It's one of the more fun parts of planning – your dreams from your vision coming to life! You can have as little or as much assistance with this as you like, and have as big or as little a budget as you need. This is the time to get creative!

For the budget route, you can buy your centerpieces in bulk on Craigslist prepackaged, just add water! Or you can simply use what you have. If you're renting a venue, does it come with certain decorations? Look around your own home for things you can use for decorations. Ask friends to loan and give you decorations. Weddings are joyous occasions and most people in your circle will be more than happy to help. Another is Christmas decorations: Christmas decorations can be repurposed for any time of season, such as clear Christmas lights, flowers, or bells. Stock up on them when they're at their cheapest – right around Thanksgiving or just after the New Year.

Of course, if your venue is already beautiful, then it won't need much money put into it for décor! Also, outdoor venues rarely need much décor. If you're worried about accessibility for outdoor venues, there are a few ways to tackle this.

Outdoor venues can be made wheelchair-accessible, so you can get the natural décor along with something unique: a wooden aisle. At an outdoor venue, wooden planks built together upon grass can form a wheelchair-accessible aisle. At most venues it's also suggested to use a bench at the altar so both partners can be eye level sitting side-by-side when one of the partners is a wheelchair user. For more accessible elegance, try using material on wheelchair-accessible ramps that fits between the user's wheels. All of these décor ideas are great for indoor or outdoor venues for accessibility.

DIY Signage

DIY signage is easy to do, especially using technology or if you're handy and have a community that's handy. I created seating charts, menus, and welcome signs in Canva. My free Canva.com account was perfect for designing classy signage for my wedding.

My family also is handy, as is my husband. They built an arbor out of juniper trees in our back yard and burned phrases onto wood to place around the venue. It took a group, but it was done.

Ordering Signage

Etsy and Minted are perfect places to order your signs. They both have everything from partial DIY to complete handmade welcome signs, seating charts, and menus, as well as cute phrasing for décor.

Favors & Gifts

Favors and gifts are a very small, personal touch on the wedding. Favors for your guests should be a reflection of who you are as a couple or your wedding's theme. Some favors do all of that and provide a function in your ceremony, such as fans on a hot day, or coffee mugs for a winter wedding. It's important to return to the vision you established at the beginning of this book for this section.

Because favors generally aren't a very memorable part of the wedding, I will point you in the direction of DollarTree.com. There you can buy in bulk to suit your theme for your wedding favors. Amazon.com also lets you buy in bulk.

Premarital Counselling

Premarital counseling is more important than you'd think. Many faith groups have premarital classes where you will meet other couples also learning communication skills like conflict resolution and budgeting. Even if you've been together a long time, marriage does change the relationship, and a brush up on relationship skills never hurts. If you're uncomfortable with a faith-based premarital counseling regimen, you can go to a regular secular counselor for premarital counseling and get a discount on your marriage license!

It's important not to do premarital counseling too early on in your engagement if you go the secular route – getting your discount on your license typically covers only 4 weeks in some states.

Accommodations

Accommodations for Yourself

Step #1. Contact the venue before the wedding and let them know your health problems and concerns. Be a s open as humanly possible. As long as you've put a deposit down and signed a contract, there's nothing to fear!

Step #2. Contact your caterer with all of your food concerns two weeks before your big day.

Step #3. Talk to your officiant. Go over your mobility concerns. Perhaps you need to sit in a decorated chair due to chronic pain during the ceremony or have a 5-minute ceremony. Go over the shortened ceremony and all of the steps (to and from the chair, who is doing what) with your officiant. If you have brain fog, let the officiant know so they can move through the vows and ceremony more slowly. Most officiants are happy to accommodate. An example of this is Stephen, who requested accommodations: "[I needed] a chair mainly. Plus the Father spoke a bit slower than usual. He knew about my health needs as we told him beforehand." He was seated for his ceremony.

Step #4: Call your doctor to devise a day-of plan. One of our contributors took extra prescription-strength medication on her wedding day. Her condition is severe and painful when she eats, so she "avoided all food and drink until the reception." She says she was symptom free the day of the wedding.

Step #5: Come up with a wedding first aid kit for your condition and designate someone in the wedding party to keep it. Tell them how to use it. This could be as simple as keeping up with your medications to something more complex.

Step #6: Working with your wedding party, devise a plan for your wedding suite at the venue for emergencies, naps during the reception, and human filters. A human filter may be someone who can speak for you or translate your thoughts and interpret for others if you are experiencing symptoms.

Making Accommodations for Yourself with Your Wedding Party

Step #1. When do I leave my wedding suite and for what reasons?

Step #2. How do I move around the ceremony and reception space? Who is with me?

Step #3. What constitutes an emergency and what should my wedding party do?

Step #4. If I have an emergency who calls or who knows how to take care of me?

Step #5. Who covers for me while I go take naps in my wedding suite or helps me get there by fending people off?

Step #6. If I am irritable because of a physical or mental condition, who is my human filter, or someone who can handle my emotions for me?

The day of the wedding can be stressful, in good ways and bad, but mostly good! Stress can cause all kinds of problems with people, whether you're disabled or not. If you are disabled, stress might impact your health more than you want it to. It's important to delegate tasks to lower symptoms and stress levels in Amy's experience. "I was still having some head cold symptoms and a fair amount of fatigue but didn't have any gut, skin, or pain flares thank goodness! Everyone was really helpful and all I had to do was ask for help if I needed it. We had already communicated well with everyone about how we wanted to keep things relaxed and enjoyable and everyone really stepped up to make that happen." With teamwork, your wedding can be happy-stress and low-stress. You will feel so much joy from your community supporting you to add to what you are already feeling in your heart.

Accommodations for Your Guests

Accommodating your guests can be straightforward. The largest part is housing out-of-town guests in hotels. There are great ways to get lower prices on hotels for your guests. Although guest accommodation was largely previously covered, we will cover how to treat difficult family members with ease.

Difficult Family Members

Maybe you have a family member who is an alcoholic or a drug addict. Or perhaps a grandparent who has a progressing case of dementia. Don't leave them sitting next to either of your parents. Find a family friend to "babysit" them for the wedding and keep them away from the immediate family and anything else that might get them into trouble.

A Note to Vendors

I reached out to my disability community to see what they would like wedding vendors to know from a disabled perspective. Some had faced discrimination, and others pure ignorance of their needs.

In order to prevent the former from keeping occurring, I wanted to find a way to communicate with vendors. So I decided to open a dialogue. My question to the contributors was, "What are three things you would want a vendor to know?"

Carrie-Ann, a wheelchair user, thinks vendors should know, "Disabled brides exist, and our requirements are personal to us. So that we can consider your venue, we need detailed, accurate accessibility information. We need to not only consider our own needs, but also those of our family and friends who may have medical conditions." She has cerebral palsy and found difficulty during her planning to find a venue.

Stephen explains more about the range of disability and the importance of vendors asking questions. "Everyone is different. Ask what makes the couple more comfortable. Disability is a myriad of symptoms. No one is affected the same. Best to ask every time." He has a host of chronic conditions, including male fibromyalgia, which is rare.

Rachel has fibromyalgia and myalgia encephalitis, AKA chronic fatigue syndrome, as well as chronic migraines. She asks vendors to stick to her plans for good reasons. "1. I have limited energy. We need to make contingency plans now, so that you can handle it on the day. 2. You will need to be flexible. My need for a 10-minute rest overrides your need to take photos or serve dinner. (I would phrase it more nicely than that!) 3. Stick to the plan. Don't 'use your initiative' and add flashing lights, or change the order of the day, or assume I changed my name and introduce us as 'Mr. and Mrs.' when we were asked to use our first names, or do anything we have not discussed. I know I sound like a control freak but there's a reason I have set things up as I have, and that is so that I can get through the day without too much pain and exhaustion." Not respecting someone's requests can lead to serious symptoms on the wedding day, and ruining your own industry.

Meagan also has two rare diseases and has general good suggestions for vendors. "One would be if there were diet restrictions that needed to be accommodated. It would be good for them to know about any mobility issues that may need to be considered for those involved or invited. And flexibility where possible such as on timing or ability to take a break from the events to allow for a rest period." She has permanent neck pain and limited mobility due to her illnesses.

Amy found wedding planning too stressful when she tried going the traditional route. "I would love wedding vendors to know how to work with a couple to create a calm, small, intimate ceremony. I didn't get the impression that I could have that with any of the vendors we looked at. There were too many details, the guest minimums were huge and it all felt too commercialized.

So I guess the three things I'd like vendors to know is that not all brides want everything 1. Overanalyzed and over-planned, 2. HUGE, and 3. Commercial. I just wanted a beautiful space where someone else took care of the decorations, I could show up in my pretty dress, commit my vows to my husband, and then kick back and enjoy celebrating with a small group of people whom I love." She ended up holding her wedding in her backyard with an intimate ceremony. Her wedding planning funds went into renovating the backyard, which was more practical in her case. Amy has hypermobile Ehlers-Danlos syndrome, or hEDs.

K. W. Warburton faced significant challenges during her wedding planning, especially when she disclosed her postural orthostatic tachy-cardia syndrome (POTS) to vendors later on in the process. "1. Not everyone is able to have a big wedding. Small weddings deserve your full attention as well. 2. Accessibility and accommodations are not op-tional and are requirements for everyone to enjoy the day. 3. Be professional. Educate yourself on your client's disability or illness to better understand their needs." The lack of professionalism on vendors' part in reaction to her POTS is a huge red flag that something needs to change in the industry.

Now the dialogue has started, and I hope this is a sign to the wedding vendor community to take notice. Not only to these answers, but perhaps this entire book. Let's begin open conversations between the disabled world and the wider population. At the very least listening to your clientele will be good for your business, I guarantee it.

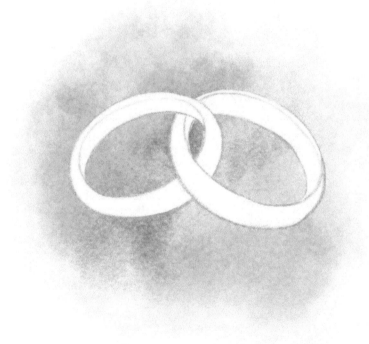

The Wedding Day

Timeline

Weddings produce all kinds of feelings. Butterflies, jitters, excitement. Here is a roadmap of your entire day from start to finish to your walk down the aisle! Please note that you may eliminate as many of these as you like. For example, we did not do a garter toss or a bouquet toss.When it comes to your wedding day timeline, Fred and Rachel suggest, "thinking about your priorities. Where do you want to expend your energy? The ceremony was the important thing for us. I wanted nice photos but I also didn't want to waste an hour's worth of energy on them, so we picked the important groups/ shots we wanted and then had a lot of more informal or reportage shots done, which was usual at the time. We didn't care about the first dance, so we rushed through that – we had about 30 seconds of us on our own and then were joined by the parents and bridal party in the same song." Rachel was able to take breaks in her suite once the dancing began. If you value the ceremony the most, invest in more rituals as outlined in the order of ceremony, and allot more time. Have a shorter reception at a place where you can retreat to your private room and lay down if you need.

The following is a timeline of how the day-of the wedding will go. Let's assume you walk down the aisle at 4pm.

10:00 am – Flowers arrive or are picked up

12:00 pm – Cake arrives

1:00 – Hair

2:00 – Makeup

3:00 – Getting into wedding dress by this point

3:30 – You are ready to go and waiting

3:30 – Videographer, photographer arrive

3:45 – Guests begin to arrive

4:00 – Couple walks down the aisle

4:30 – Ceremony ends

4:40 – Pictures with family photoshoot begins, beginning of cocktail hour

5:40 – Grand Entry, couple is announced

5:45 – Dinner is served

6:30 – Cut the cake

6:45 – Dance floor officially open

7:45 – Bouquet Toss

7:50 – Garter Toss

8:00 – Partying resumes

10:00pm – Grand Exit and Sendoff

You can walk down the aisle and plan your day around it any way you like. Take a cue from K. W. Warburton, who told me, "I planned the day to minimize symptoms. I arranged to have the ceremony at 2 pm, a time when I am most alert and my morning meds have kicked in. I also sat down for my vows, which I thought would ruin the photos, but they turned out great!" There are no rules, just ideas. Do what is right for you. It's your day!

Order of Ceremony

The Order of Ceremony tells you how the wedding happens, goes down, or how you end up married. All of your planning has taken you to this point, and it's going to be awesome.

Wedding ceremonies can be as complex or simple as you wish. This is a simple outline that you can cross off what you don't want to get an idea of what your day will look like. You can eliminate 40% of this list to have a short ceremony if your symptoms make it difficult to stand for long periods of time, or you merely want to get it over quickly. Keep in mind what you want and need as you go through this outline. You can change up certain parts – such as dancing through the processional – and having a quirky unity ceremony to make your day more fun.

- Prelude
- Seating of the Grandparents (may or may not be ushered by ushers or wedding party attendants)
- Seating of the Parents (may or may not be ushered by ushers or wedding party attendants)
- Processional
- Welcome
- Opening prayer

- Reading #1
- Ritual
    - Unity candle
    - Sand mixing
    - Handfasting
    - Make up your own!
- Reading 2
- Song or Instrumental Music
- Declaration of Intention
- Exchange of Vows
- Blessing of Rings
- Exchange of Rings
- Marriage Blessing
- Declaration of Marriage
- First Kiss
- Presentation of the Couple
- Recessional
- Receiving line

It's really that simple! Wedding ceremonies are really straight lines. You will be wonderful! Remember to have fun. Enjoy the moment and take mental photographs. No matter if anything goes wrong, it's still the perfect, best day – you have found your person, and they have found you.

Remember, it's a love story!

You deserve to be loved, and you are loved. If you're reading this, someone loves you, somewhere in this world. Feel it. There are some real love stories involving disability and that love shines with it, not necessarily in spite of it. K. W. Warburton's real love story about developing postural orthostatic tachycardia syndrome (POTS) during her engagement is proof that weddings really are about the love story. "My husband and I met in our first year and he proposed after just 6 months (he was 18, I was 19). My husband was on a three-year course and I was on a four-year course. We had always planned to get married the year after I graduated from university. However, I developed POTS in my final year and became bedridden almost instantly, so we decided to postpone our wedding until I was well again. When I found out that I had a long-term chronic illness, we had to make a decision on when and how we would like to get married. We decided that we didn't want to wait any longer, as we had been engaged for almost 5 years at that point. We scaled down our wedding plans and I started physiotherapy so that I would be able to walk down the aisle." Your wedding exists with your disability. So does your love. Celebrate it!

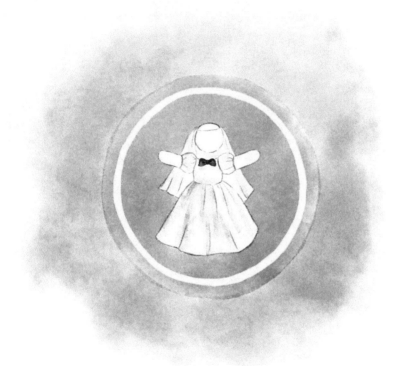

Planning with Your Disabled Partner

A Resource for You

How Sweet It Is to be Loved…

Congratulations! You have found your person. Perhaps this is why you picked up this book – you don't know how to plan a wedding around their needs and yours.

I'm here to tell you that it's hard but it's possible. Like all matters in love, it is high-risk, high-payoff, and your relationship during wedding planning would be no different if your partner was able-bodied.

Your relationship changes during wedding planning. One of you might try to power play too much – whether that's you or your partner depends on how the relationship goes, but it's still something to watch for. What should you do if that happens? Take a step back, breathe, and remember we're all human.

Of course, there is always the dynamic of inequality when it comes to the planning burdens. Wedding planning isn't always a balanced 50/50 team sport between partners. Sometimes it's 60/40, 80/20 or, at its worst … 0/100.

Communicate openly with your partner and use some of the guides in this book where needed, and happy planning! We hope we've made the experience smoother for you with our work.

Love,

Meara Bartlett

A Note from Your Partner

As a disabled partner, there are only a few things I want my able-bodied partner to know: I love you, I'm sorry I don't always show it well, and I do try even if it seems lacking. I'm sure you think the same thoughts sometimes about how you feel toward your disabled partner. You're two humans about to be in this forever. Remember the human part as we both struggle a little with our new phase of connection, and we'll be fine.

Wedding planning is about communication and connection. Remembering that wedding planning is a team sport, and including me, your disabled partner, is important. When Stephen remembers his wedding planning life season it was "50/50" responsibility-wise and his wife did "most of the calling." He expressed gratitude for what his wife did during the process and that he only wished one thing was different. Your disabled partner is thankful for you, whether they are able to communicate it well or not, or you are able to sense it well or not. This is all part of your new phase of connection.

How to Feel About Your Partner's Involvement

There are many types of wedding planners in this world. I planned every little detail in three months before grad school started and I was diagnosed with a tentative "Possible fibromyalgia with a dash of lupus and rheumatoid arthritis jumbalaya?" With my wedding, I hit the ground running. But I wanted support from my partner. We still had months to go to our big day, and I felt alone after my medical emergencies. It seemed to me he didn't care. Once, he even refused to speak to the day-of coordinator!

But wedding planning does not predict a marriage. It doesn't reflect on who your partner will be as a spouse. Close those articles written by supposed fortune tellers about how wedding vendors could tell when such and such a poor person was headed for divorce.

My wedding planning may have been 0/100, but I gained a loving, caring spouse who cleans the tub, is building a rose garden for me, does the dishes, and lets me cry. There is really nothing more a person can ask for when you factor in what humanity means.

Now, let's talk about your disabled partner. Disabled people of all kinds have limited energy reserves. A unit of energy is called a spoon. When a person completes an action or feels an intense emotion, a spoon is taken by the spoon gods. This is called the Spoon Theory by Christine Miserandino, referenced in the Introduction. Your partner is probably just as stressed as you are if they are checking out. Because of all the stress they're caught up in, precious spoons of energy are being wasted. Instead of snapping at you because they're tired, they may avoid the wedding subject altogether.

If you find yourself absolutely drowning, consider having premarital couples counseling to improve your communication and find out what's going on with your partner. Or, play the trading game – for every wedding thing your partner does, you take a load off of their plate.

Don't panic if this doesn't work. People with spoons, or spoonies, have smaller boundaries than able-bodied people do. We have to be this way in order to function and be decently kind. Your partner may not want to risk the relationship for the wedding planning.

Rachel's Story

When talking about stressors and support, Rachel had a few words about the obstacles and love she encountered in her wedding planning journey. "The biggest stress was family politics. The second biggest stress was whether or not I would be physically well on the day, and whether I would have the stamina to get through it. My mum, husband and I were all concerned about that. In the end, I did get through it, mostly on adrenaline, and didn't realize how much pain I was in until we got to the hotel that night.

The biggest support was that my husband understood my illness and limitations, and wasn't going to feel upset if everything didn't go perfectly. He was very supportive and I knew that, as long as I got through the ceremony, if I was exhausted at the reception then he wouldn't be upset."

As someone else who occasionally has to use a cane and had this same experience, I understood Rachel when she explained "I can walk without my walking stick and it was important to me that I didn't use it to walk down the aisle. Someone had it in their car in case I needed it at the reception. I remember just being exhausted after the ceremony, and there's a photo of me resting my head on my husband's chest as we waited to sign the register. I had planned to rest in the car on the way to the reception venue but we were just too excited. However, that level of understanding from my husband was vital." I leaned over the counter as my husband, father and I signed our wedding license. Throughout most of my wedding, I was leaning on a wall or my husband as I forwent my cane.

My husband tried his hardest to understand what I went through. During our engagement, he drove 45 minutes twice a week to hold my hand at my bedside. He is never angry when we go on walks together and I have to rest, and even encourages me to use my mobility aids.

What I have to say here is that understanding and respect are the core of love, and they will take you through wedding planning with your disabled partner.

Thank You for Reading

Thank you for reading. Without you, I could not have authored this book. We all must stick together. I know that without you, I would not have known I wasn't alone, and that there wasn't someone who might have needed someone to tell them to be brave in the face of prejudice, like I once did. Or someone to tell them that their wedding would be wonderful, no matter what happens, that had had struggles similar to theirs.

I want you to know that you are beautiful and perfect just the way you are. The way you came into this world or the way you became is divine. Remember, you deserve this, no matter what the world might have told you, or you have told yourself. You are captivating. It's tough out there, but now you won't have to go it alone.

Everything you have ever been through has brought you to this point. Every time you've ever felt small is about to have a celebration. It has all been worth it in the end, and it always will be.

Every person you have ever been has led you to the lovely human being you are. Never forget this, my friend.

All roads lead to the same wonderful place, and here you are reading this book, which is all for you.

Congratulations!

Meara Bartlett

Helpful Resources

Allseated.com

Amazon.com

Canva.com

CustomCurvyBride.com

DavidsBridal.com

DesireeMarieDesign.com

DollarTree.com

Etsy.com

Google Drive, Drive.Google.com

Google Sheets, Sheets.Google.com

Minted.com

OffbeatBride.com

Shutterfly.com

TheKnot.com

TheMighty.com

Thumbtack.com

WeddingWire.com

Works Cited

Anonymous, Amy. Personal Interview. 3 April 2020.

Anonymous, Meagan. Personal Interview. 29 May 2020.

Anonymous, Rachel. Personal Interview. 29 March 2020.

Anonymous, Stephen. Personal Interview. 5 May 2020.

Duhon, Cyndee. "7 Ways to Make Your Wedding
    Accessible." *MobilityWorks*, 16 May 2019, www.mobilityworks.
    com/blog/7-ways-to-make-your-wedding-accessible/amp/.

Fleming, Carrie-Ann. "Disabled Weddings: How to Plan an
    Accessible Day." *The Guardian*, Guardian News and Media,
    17 Feb. 2012, www.theguardian.com/lifeandstyle/2012/feb/17/
    disabled-weddings-plan-accessible-day.

Jenny. *Life's a Polyp*, 1 Jan. 2020, www.lifesapolyp.com/.
@LifesaPolyp.

Lightley, Carrie-Ann. "Carrie-Ann Lightley: Disabled Blogger and
    Travel Writer." *Carrieannlightley*, www.carrieannlightley.com/.

Lightley, Carrie-Ann. Personal Interview. 28 April 2020.

Miserandino, Christine. "The Spoon Theory." *But You Don't Look
    Sick? Support for Those with Invisible Illness or Chronic Illness*, 26
    Apr. 2013, butyoudontlooksick.com/articles/written-by-christine/the-
    spoon-theory/.

Offbeat Bride, 19 June 2020, offbeatbride.com/.

Jess. *Study In Fitness*. studyinfitness.com/.

    @StudyInFitness

Warburton, K. W. Personal Interview. 6 April 2020.

Warburton, K W. *The Reluctant Spoonie*, 6 Jan. 2020,

    thereluctantspoonie.com/.

    @TheReluctantSpoonie

CPSIA information can be obtained
at www.ICGtesting.com
Printed in the USA
LVHW060002060221
678489LV00003B/34